André Serra
Sandra Sardinha
Roberto Azevedo

Cleft lip and palate - Alveolar bone grafts

André Serra
Sandra Sardinha
Roberto Azevedo

Cleft lip and palate - Alveolar bone grafts

The challenge of rehabilitation for cleft patients

ScienciaScripts

Imprint

Any brand names and product names mentioned in this book are subject to trademark, brand or patent protection and are trademarks or registered trademarks of their respective holders. The use of brand names, product names, common names, trade names, product descriptions etc. even without a particular marking in this work is in no way to be construed to mean that such names may be regarded as unrestricted in respect of trademark and brand protection legislation and could thus be used by anyone.

Cover image: www.ingimage.com

This book is a translation from the original published under ISBN 978-613-9-66349-1.

Publisher:
Sciencia Scripts
is a trademark of
Dodo Books Indian Ocean Ltd. and OmniScriptum S.R.L publishing group

120 High Road, East Finchley, London, N2 9ED, United Kingdom
Str. Armeneasca 28/1, office 1, Chisinau MD-2012, Republic of Moldova, Europe
Printed at: see last page
ISBN: 978-620-8-02055-2

SUMMARY

SUMMARY:

Alveolar bone grafting is a standard procedure for occlusal, aesthetic and functional rehabilitation of patients with cleft lip and palate. The use of this technique allows for the re-establishment of maxillary continuity, enabling tooth eruption and movement through the formation of a bone bridge. Its varied success rate is related to systemic, surgical and sociocultural factors. This study will assess the success rate of alveolar bone grafts carried out at the Centrinho do Hospital Santo Antônio in Salvador-BA, between January 2013 and December 2014. Data from the medical records of the sample population will be used, as well as clinical examination and evaluation of radiographic examinations. Epidemiological data will be correlated with the success rates of this procedure in order to establish the possible causes of poor bone formation and graft loss.

CHAPTER 1

INTRODUCTION

Cleft lip and palate are considered to be the most common congenital facial disorders worldwide. In Brazil, they occur at a rate of 1:650 (CARLINI *et al,* 2000). Statistically, in 2012 a total of 1,524 occurrences of these malformations were recorded in Datasus, 336 of which were in the northeast region. The prevalence of cleft lip and palate in the Northeast is 9.72/1 Omil live births, and for cleft palate 2.41/1 Omil live births (COUTINHO et *al,* 2009).

From its Latin etymology, the word "fissure" means crack, opening. Biologically, it is defined as a "solution of continuity" and in the pathological context it denotes any innate anatomical opening that deviates from normal (SILVA FILHO *et al,* 2007). Chronologically, these malformations are established early in intrauterine life, through morphological alterations at 8ª and 12ª weeks (LE et *al,* 2009). Their aetiology is multifactorial and consists of the interrelation of genetic, environmental and cultural factors. Around 70 per cent occur in isolation, although they can be associated with other anomalies (BRYDON et *al,* 2014). The most frequent anomalies are in the facial region (21 per cent), the eye (17 per cent), the central nervous system (15 per cent), the gastrointestinal tract (3 per cent) and the urogenital tract (2 per cent) (SEKHON et *al,* 2011).

As an important step in the rehabilitation of patients with cleft lip and palate, alveolar bone grafting surgery is aimed at prosthetic rehabilitation through adequate local bone volume (LE et *al,* 2009). A variety of factors can interfere with its outcome, contributing to its success rate. Conditions such as age, stage of tooth eruption, size of the cleft and the patient's systemic conditions, as well as the quantity and quality of the soft tissue to cover the graft and the surgical technique used make it difficult to define a prognosis (BORBA et al, 2013).

Alveolar bone grafting is based on the stages of tooth development and is thus classified as primary, secondary or tertiary (FREITAS et al, 2012). Its role is to provide support for the alar base and nasal symmetry, eliminate oronasal fistulas, increase maxillary stability, allow tooth eruption and orthodontic movement and enable prosthetic rehabilitation (PRECIOUS DS, 2009). Secondary grafting is the most commonly used technique in cleft alveolar reconstruction procedures. Several studies have shown the effectiveness of this procedure and its relationship with the growth of the middle third of the face (SANTIAGO et al, 2014)(BORBA et al, 2013)(HALL et al, 1983).

As for the type of material used to fill the cleft, some situations can change the choice. The size and volume of bone required, the presence of teeth, the recovery of the donor site and systemic factors will indicate the best material to use (KAZEMI et al, 2002). Autogenous bone is currently the gold standard in alveolar reconstruction for cleft patients, and its good availability and low cost favour its use (THUAKSUBAM et al, 2010). However, high rates of bone resorption have been found in the literature. In a study by Tai et al. (2000), a volume loss of approximately 43.1% was found after one year's follow-up with cone beam tomography, while Feichtinger et al. in 2006 reported a bone loss of more than 49.5%. Criteria such as type of cleft, time of bone grafting, oral hygiene care, make it difficult to predict success and failure rates related to the rehabilitation of patients with cleft lip and palate.

CHAPTER 2

OBJECTIVE

2.1 General Objective

To evaluate the success rate of alveolar bone grafts performed at a reference centre in Bahia between January 2013 and December 2014.

2.2 Specific objectives

- To assess bone formation in the alveolar fissure using periapical radiography;

- Relate epidemiological data to graft success rates.

CHAPTER 3

LITERATURE REVIEW

3.1 Facial development

In order to better understand the occurrence of cleft lip and palate, it is necessary to understand craniofacial development. The formation of the head and neck, according to Moore et al. (1990), basically consists of the development of the branchial apparatus. It consists of gill arches, pharyngeal pouches, gill slits and gill membranes.

Most congenital malformations in this region originate during the structural transformations that take place in the branchial apparatus. The branchial arches begin to develop at the beginning of the 4th week[a] as cells of the neural crest migrate to the region of the future head and neck. The 1st branchial arch, the primordium of the mandible, appears as a slight elevation of the lateral surface of the pharynx in formation. [a]By the end of the 4th week, four pairs of gill arches are visible in the external plane, separated from each other by the gill slits (SILVA, 1999).

From this stage, the frontonasal protrusion, the pair of maxillary protrusions and a pair of mandibular protrusions are formed. The first forms the glabella, the dorsum and apex of the nose. The lateral nasal protrusions form the wings of the nose, while the medial nasal protrusions form, among other structures, the nasal septum (AVERY, 2001)(MOORE, PERSAUD, 2008).

The maxillary protrusions give rise to the upper cheeks, the maxilla and a large part of the upper lip. In contrast, the mandibular protrusions form the lower lip, mandible, lower cheeks and chin (MOORE, PERSAUD, 2008). During the sixth week of development, the maxillary and mandibular tissues fuse. The upper lip is then formed by the junction of the medial nasal process and two lateral maxillary segments (SILVA FILHO, FREITAS, 2007).

The medial nasal process is in close contact with the medial face of the maxillary process, and the lateral nasal process is above it. Clefts of the lip and maxillary alveolus, whether unilateral or bilateral, can occur due to a lack of fusion between the medial nasal process and the maxillary processes (AVERY, 2001). The palate is formed from the primary palate and secondary palate. [a]The primary palate develops at the end of the 5th week and houses the incisor teeth of the maxilla, giving rise to the anterior part of the incisor foramen. The secondary palate is the primordium of the hard and soft parts of the palate and extends posteriorly from this foramen. Therefore, pre-foramen incisor malformations and post-foramen incisor malformations are embryologically distinct. Until the 3rd month of gestation, the hard and soft palates are completely isolated from the oral and nasal cavities (SILVA, 1999).

At the end of the 6th week[a] the lips and gums begin to form. [a]During the 7th week of intrauterine life, the lateral processes of the palate lodge and move to a horizontal position above the tongue. They approach and merge at the midline. They also fuse with the primary palate and the nasal septum. This fusion begins anteriorly during the 9th week[a] and is completed posteriorly, in the region of the uvula, around the 12th week[a] (SILVA, 1999)(SILVA FILHO, FREITAS, 2007)(MOORE, PERSAUD, 2008).

Cleft palates can occur due to a lack of fusion between these structures, and the most critical period of palatogenesis is from the end of the sixth week to the beginning of the ninth week, completing only in the twelfth week of development (MOORE, PERSAUD, 2008).

3.2 Etiology, Epidemiology of Cleft Lip and Palate

Cleft lip and palate are considered to be the most common congenital facial disorders in the world. In Brazil, they occur at a rate of 1:650 births and there are an estimated 225,000 people with these lesions in the country (CARLINI *et al,* 2000). The frequency of these alterations is higher in Orientals and lower in blacks, with a male/female ratio of 3:2. The most affected structure in men is the lip and in women the palate and three quarters of affected patients have unilateral clefts (CARLINI et *al,* 2000).

Individuals with unfavourable socioeconomic status are at greater risk of suffering from cleft lip and palate (CERQUEIRA et *al,* 2005). This factor influences people's state of health and there may be a lack of access to the necessary care, such as prenatal care and access to a diet composed of the nutrients necessary for the proper development of the foetus (CERQUEIRA et *al,* 2005)(ESCOFFIÉ-RAMÍREZ et *al,* 2010)(GARIB et *al,* 2010).

Its aetiology is still controversial, but it may be associated with genetic and environmental factors, among others. Genetic factors are generally associated with syndromes. Environmental factors are related to smoking, excessive alcohol consumption, the use of anticonvulsant drugs, ionising radiation, nutritional and infectious factors, which occur during the embryonic and early foetal periods (COUTINHO *et al,* 2009). Some agents, such as teratogenic drugs, also increase a mother's risk of conceiving a child with cleft lip and palate. Other studies have found a correlation between the age of the parents and the incidence of clefts (BARONEZA et *al,* 2005).

Cleft lip and palate cause various alterations that compromise speech, aesthetics, dental positioning, swallowing, phonation, breathing and nutrition (FIGUEIREDO et *al*, 2008), and can also cause hearing impairment due to recurrent otitis media (ZAMBONATO et *al*, 2009). The maxillomandibular relationship can become unfavourable due to dental alterations, such as the presence of extranumerary teeth, fusion, dental agenesis, thus causing various malocclusions (FIGUEIREDO et *al*, 2008)(MASTRANTONIO, CASTILHO, CARRARA, 2009).

3.3 Classification of cracks

The first widely accepted classification system was that of Kernahan and Stark in 1958. This described the most common cleft lip and palate using a system of symbols. Seeking to describe unusual types of cleft, Kernahan in 1971 used a symbolic scheme using the letter "Y". This modification had some shortcomings and was later modified by Millard in 1977 (KHAN et al, 2013).

Several classifications are used for cleft lip and palate, but few have clinical application. Davis and Ritchie's (1922) classification is based on the position of the cleft in relation to the alveolar process. In group I, the cleft is pre-alveolar when it involves only the lip. It can be unilateral, bilateral or median. Group II has a post-alveolar cleft, involving the soft palate, soft palate plus hard palate or submucous cleft and group III has trans-alveolar clefts, which can be unilateral, bilateral or median. Veau (1931) used yet another system that divided cleft lip and palate patients into four types. Type I had clefts of the soft palate, type II had clefts of the hard palate and soft palate up to the incisive foramen, type III had clefts of the hard palate and soft palate up to the incisive foramen in the midline, extending to the alveolus in the position of the future lateral incisor tooth on one side. Type IV had a complete bilateral cleft (KHAN et al, 2013).

Kernahan and Stark (1958) and Harkins (1962) proposed classifications that were adopted by the American Cleft Palate Association. Seeking to standardise and accurately describe the types, location and extent of cleft lip and palate deformities, the scientific community sought to create more clinical classification parameters. In addition to facilitating understanding and scientific documentation, the aim of this system was to overcome language barriers and enable standardised computer analysis (KHAN et al, 2013).

Clefts can have varying degrees of severity depending on their presentation, and can be unilateral or bilateral, complete or incomplete and rare. The most widely used classification is that of Spina (1974) and takes the incisive foramen as the reference point. They can be classified as a pre-foramen incisor cleft, where it exclusively affects the lip due to a lack of fusion between the maxillary processes and the median nasal processes. It can be unilateral, bilateral or median and complete or incomplete. It is complete when there are small indentations in the mucosa of the vermilion and/or skin of the lip and total rupture of the lip and alveolar ridge, passing through the floor of the nose and ending at the incisive foramen. When this type of cleft does not involve the alveolar ridge, there are no dental anomalies. The nasal tip is deflected towards the non-cracked side. Post-incisive foramen cleft characterised by cleft palates, resulting from the lack of fusion of the palatine processes with each other and with the nasal septum. They are median and can affect only the uvula, soft palate (incomplete) or involve the hard palate (complete). This type of cleft is not as aesthetically pleasing as others, but it does lead to a nasal resonance of speech due to the inadequate function of the velopharyngeal mechanism. This is the cleft that is most often associated with other congenital defects. The mildest form of this cleft has a bifid uvula and does not always require a therapeutic approach. Transforamen incisor cleft, resulting from non-fusion of the mesenchyme of the lateral palatine processes of the palate and nasal septum. It affects the lip, alveolar arch and the entire palate. It can be unilateral or bilateral and complete or incomplete (when only the lip is unaffected), the most severe form. Rare facial clefts involve the lips, nose, eyes and jaw. There are also submucosal clefts which have a deficiency of muscle tissue (soft palate) or bone (hard palate) beneath the intact mucous layer, giving a false idea of normality. The most obvious sign is located on the midline of the palate, which will be much lighter in colour than the rest of the mucosa. It is often associated with the presence of a bifid uvula and hypernasality of speech. The symptom that babies with this type of cleft present is the escape of milk through the nose (BRUNER *et al*, 2012).

Altmann et *al*. (1997) reported the existence of an occult submucosal fissure that can only be visualised through nasofibroscopy and consists of hypoplasia of the uvula muscle and diastasis of the velar muscles on the nasal surface (BRUNER et *al*, 2012).

3.4 Surgical protocols

Following the operational standards developed at the University of São Paulo's Craniofacial Anomalies Rehabilitation Hospital, one of the main primary roles in the treatment of patients with cleft lip and palate is surgical repair to re-establish eating, speech and cosmetic changes (SHKOUKANI et *al*, 2013).

Treatment should begin with reparative plastic surgery, known as cheiloplasty (lip surgery) and palatoplasty (palate surgery) (TUJI et *al*, 2009). Cheiloplasty is often performed in the third month of life, but results in a rigid, fibrous lip "band", which prevents proper maxillary growth, resulting in maxillofacial anomalies (LURENTT et *al,* 2012).

The aim of surgical correction of cleft lip is to restore continuity to the orbicularis oris muscle in order to provide functionality to the lip, as well as to achieve an anatomically and aesthetically normal lip. Various techniques have been described for lip correction, including the Millard technique (RASPALL, 1997). This technique uses downward rotation of the superiorly displaced middle segment of the lip with advancement of the lateral lip flap to correct the defect below the nose. This technique produces minimal tissue loss, creates a suture line consistent with the filter on the cleft side, preserves the cupid's bow, repositions the base of the nasal ala and provides tension to reduce nasal widening, guides construction of the nasal base, and is extremely versatile for the type of cleft the surgeon may encounter (SHKOUKANI *et al,* 2013).

Most patients who have not had primary rhinoplasty have significantly more severe nasal deformities and functional disorders, which can be explained by growth alterations caused by the primary intervention. The more severe the deformity, the more severe the asymmetry and the worse the nasal airflow and functional disorders. For this reason, primary rhinoplasty is recommended at the same time as primary lip restoration (ANNASTASSOV, JOOS, 2001).

Between the ages of 12 months, cleft palate is usually corrected by palatoplasty. This procedure is used to correct the functional and aesthetic limitations resulting from this malformation (AMORIM, 2014). Its aim is to create a correct swallowing mechanism, pharyngeal velamentum, without interfering with the growth of the mid-facial third

(RASPALL, 1997).

The Von Langenbeck palatoplasty is the oldest technique still in use and consists of closing the palate by approximating its margins, facilitated by making a lateral incision along the maxillary tuberosity up to the posterior portion of the alveolar ridge. This technique is responsible for maxillary hypoplasia, with retromaxilia and dental malocclusion (AMORIM, 2014).

Secondary surgeries of the lip or palate, lengthening of the nasal columella or even pharyngoplasties are performed from the age of six. These are useful for correcting defects and alterations that are still present after the first procedures (TUJI *et al*, 2009).

3.4.1 Alveolar Bone Grafting Technique

The alveolar process bone defect is an abnormality that affects approximately 3 out of 4 patients with cleft lip and palate (ANDERSEN et *al*, 2014). Its correction aims to provide stability to the maxillary arch, provide periodontal support to the teeth adjacent to the cleft, promote closure of the oronasal fistula, favour speech development and improve the aesthetic result (KOH et *al*, 2013).

The graft is used to correct the alveolar bone defect in pre-foramen and transforamen incisive clefts and to achieve union between the palatine processes (RIBEIRO, LEAL, THUIN, 2007). In order for people with cleft lip and palate to receive appropriate surgical treatment, protocols have been established which include everything from pre-surgical assessment to post-surgical follow-up (LIMA et *al*, 2008).

The permanence of this defect results in oronasal fistulas that promote fluid reflux during feeding, speech and jaw development disorders, lack of bone support and facial asymmetry (ANDERSEN *et al*, 2014). The alveolar bone graft technique is widely accepted as the main form of treatment and enables complete closure of the alveolar cleft.

In the study by Boyne and Sands (1972), this technique was classified according to the patient's age into: 1) primary bone graft: performed on patients under 2 years of age; 2) early secondary bone graft: performed between 2 and 5 years of age; 3) secondary bone graft: between 6 and 15 years of age, and 4) late bone graft: on individuals with complete bone and tooth formation (FREITAS et *al*, 2012).

Silva Filho et *al* (1992) modified this classification, relating it to the stage of tooth development. Thus, the graft was categorised into: 1) primary bone graft: performed on children up to 1 year of age, together with lip and palate repair surgery; 2) secondary bone graft: performed during the mixed dentition, subdivided into: a) early: 5 to 6 years; b) secondary: from 8 to 12 years, c) late: performed after the eruption of the permanent canine, and 3) tertiary bone graft: applied in adults (FREITAS et *al*, 2012).

Primary alveolar grafting is currently out of favour, as studies show that it impairs maxillary growth (KOH et *al*, 2013)(FREITAS et *al*, 2012). Secondary bone grafting is the most widely used technique in the reconstruction procedure. Several studies have shown its effectiveness and its relationship with the growth of the middle third of the face (SANTIAGO *et al*, 2014)(BORBA *et al*, 2013)(HALL *et al*, 1983).

Pre-surgical orthodontic treatment is fundamental in the rehabilitation of cleft patients. Orthodontic therapy is planned in separate phases, one pre- and one post-bone grafting. The poor growth of the maxilla and the alterations found in the alveolar bone are factors taken into account when planning orthodontic treatment (LIMA et *al*, 2008).

However, treatment is not restricted to surgical and orthodontic interventions alone; it also requires numerous other procedures to be carried out by professionals from different areas, as established by Ordinance 62 SAS/MS (1994), thus forming a multi-professional health care team for cleft individuals (LIMA et *al*, 2008).

3.5Bone Substitutes

Enemark et al. in 2010 argued that patients with symptomatic oronasal fistulae, lack of bone structure to enable eruption and dental support next to the fissure and who require orthodontic treatment should undergo alveolar bone grafting (ANDERSEN et *al*, 2014). As for the type of material used to fill the cleft, certain situations can change the choice. The size and volume of bone required, the presence of teeth, the recovery of the donor site and systemic factors will indicate the best material to use (KAZEMI et *al*, 2002).

Autogenous bone is currently the gold standard in alveolar reconstruction for cleft patients, and its good availability and low cost favour its use (THUAKSUBAM et *al*, 2010). It has the potential to combine all the main positive incorporation factors: osteoconduction, osteoinduction, osteogenesis and absence of immunological reaction (TANAKA et *al*, 2008)(SILVA FILHO et *al*, 2009). The advantages of autogenous bone include biocompatibility, the presence of osteogenic cells and osseoinduction (BORSTLAP et *al*, 1990) (TANAKA et *al*, 2008)(SILVA FILHO et *al*, 2009). On the other hand, a disadvantage is its known resorption potential, which can vary between 24 and 51 per cent after the first year (FEICHTINGER et *al*, 2007)(THUAKSUBAN et *al*, 2010). Some authors have observed up to 50% volume loss in the first year of follow-up (LE, WOO et *al*, 2009).

Patients who need a large amount of bone for reconstruction can opt for the removal of grafts from the iliac crest, parietal bone and tibia. The iliac crest is the most cost-effective donor site and is the most suitable for large cortico-medullary or purely medullary grafts, its main advantage being the large volume obtained (MENDONÇA et *al*, 2011)(ANDERSEN et *al*, 2014). However, it causes a great deal of morbidity and can cause complications such as fractures, seromas, sensory and gait disorders and perforations of the peritoneum (ANDERSEN et *al*, 2014).

The use of bio-material has been described in the literature and has been widely accepted over the years (LE, WOO *et al*, 2009). A clinical and radiographic study of alveolar grafts using autogenous bone and its association with an alloplastic material (Bio-oss) showed better bone formation and less morbidity in patients who received both materials, but at the end of follow-up there was a loss of bone volume in both groups (THUAKSUBAM et *al*, 2010).

The rhBMP-2 molecule is one of the alternatives for avoiding the use of bone from the iliac crest (COOTS, 2012). Considered a human recombinant bone morphogenetic protein, it is capable of inducing bone formation when placed in a suitable medium and acts by concentrating the host mesenchymal cells at the site, influencing their differentiation into osteoblasts (CHEN et *al*, 2004). Surgeries using rhBMP-2 have been carried out at HRAC-USP and the results have been as good as iliac crest grafts. The aim is to eliminate surgical morbidity and dependence on other medical professionals, making treatment simpler and more accessible. The use of rhBMP-2 has the advantages of post-operative recovery, as well as eliminating the need for a donor area and a second surgical team; however, it brings with it a major challenge in its application in public health services, due to its extremely high cost (PALONE et *al*, 2013).

3.6 Clinical and Radiographic Criteria for Success

The evaluation of success criteria in alveolar grafting is related to clinical and radiographic aspects. The absence of bone exposure, an infectious process and good tissue healing do not always indicate successful reconstruction. However, favourable imaging findings mostly lead to clinical aspects of good tissue healing (LUQUE-MARTIN *et al*, 2014).

The assessment of the bone volume obtained after grafting in the alveolar cleft is of fundamental importance. In most situations, the height and width of the bone obtained is assessed using periapical and panoramic radiographs, while its thickness can be assessed by palpation, inspection or tomography (MENDONÇA et *al*, 2011).

Radiographic criteria for assessing the success rate of alveolar bone grafts are related to the restoration of bone height and width at the level of the cleft (TABRIZI et *al*, 2013). Serial radiographic evaluations can show the amount of bone obtained during alveolar reconstruction and infer the rate of postoperative resorption, helping the surgeon to predict surgical success (NIGHTINGALE et *al*, 2003).

In a study that sought to assess the success rate of alveolar bone grafts using autogenous bone mixed with alloplastic material (hydroxyapatite), Carlini et al. (2000) used periapical radiographs to measure the bone level obtained during alveolar reconstruction. After a period of six months, the surgical results were evaluated and a bone loss of less than 3mm between the alveolar Christian and the graft was considered a success.

Relating these figures to the final result, it was also observed that the group containing a mixture of autogenous bone and alloplastic material (hydroxyapatite) had an 80 per cent success rate, while the patients who underwent reconstruction with iliac Christian had 46.7 per cent (CARLINI *et al*, 2000).

Other studies, which monitored radiographs and associated their results with the success rate of alveolar bone grafting, used standardised scales to assess bone formation in the cleft region. They observed that the procedure carried out before canine eruption increased success rates, emphasising the use of the Berglang and Chelsea scales as important tools for assessing surgical results (TRINDADE et *al*, 2005)(SHARMA et *al*, 2012).

Both scales assess the level of bone formed after alveolar reconstruction with grafts. The Berglang scale, considered the gold standard in these measurements, considers the height of the bone septum formed from the presence of the dental elements neighbouring the defect and is subdivided into 4 types. Type I shows bone gain above the amelodentine junction; in Type II the height is at least three quarters of normal height, in Type III its height is below three quarters of normal and Type IV shows no bone continuity *and* indicates total failure of the technique (TRINDADE et *al*, 2005)(SHARMA et *al*, 2012).

With the evolution of image processing, the use of computerised tomography makes it the most accurate method for evaluation. Cone beam CT scans produce information on the size of the cleft and three-dimensionally reproduce the bone volume acquired after alveolar bone grafting. This information makes it possible to accurately quantify the real gain in bone tissue and the areas of the defect that were unsuccessful (LEITE *et al*, 2014).

Pre-operative measurement of the shape and size of the bone defect is very useful for successful bone grafting. Some recent studies have reported on the relationship between preoperative measurement of the size of the bone defect using cone beam computed tomography and the actual amount of bone grafted. Through cone beam computed tomography and its 3D reconstructions, it is possible to visualise the full extent and depth of the gap, facilitating surgical planning and assessing the success rate (LEITE et *al*, 2014).

CHAPTER 4

METHODOLOGY

4.1 Study design

A longitudinal observational study was carried out of 76 patients treated at Centrinho, located at Hospital Santo Antônio, Salvador-BA, between January 2013 and December 2014. Information was collected from 53 patients who met the eligibility criteria and for this reason no sample calculation was used. This study was submitted to the Human Research Ethics Committee of the Santo Antônio Hospital (Obras Sociais Irmã Dulce) and was approved according to the criteria required by Resolution 466/2012 of the National Health Council (Annex 2).

4.2 Eligibility criteria

Patients who did not sign the Informed Consent Form (ICF) and, in the case of minors, the Informed Consent Form (ICF) were excluded from the study.

Patients who did not return for a clinical and radiographic examination, had poorly completed medical records, had had more than one alveolar grafting procedure carried out during this period and had some systemic disorder were excluded. Those with median fissures, those with syndromes and those requiring premaxillary repositioning were also removed from the sample.

4.3 Data collection procedure

The medical records of patients who met the inclusion criteria had their data collected on a form (APPENDIX A) and then tabulated in the Excel®2013 programme. This form did not contain the participant's personal details, and they were identified only by their hospital record and form number. This clinical instrument included information on the age at which the graft was performed, gender, type of cleft, oral hygiene conditions, infection rate, post-operative follow-up period and the need for surgical re-exploration.

The participants were divided according to the type of bone grafting technique used, primary, secondary or tertiary. They were also separated into 12 to 18 months and 19 to 24 months post-operatively.

The clinical examination was carried out at least one year after the graft and lasted a maximum of 10 minutes, observing the presence of a fistula and the absence of oronasal secretion.

The radiographic examination used was an analogue periapical radiograph of the cleft region at least one year after surgery. To assess bone formation, the radiographic examinations were carried out on the same radiographic apparatus and assessed by two calibrated examiners using the Bergland scale (ANNEX B).

The Berglang scale, considered the gold standard in these measurements, considers the height of the bone septum formed from the presence of the dental elements neighbouring the defect and is subdivided into 4 types. Type I shows bone gain above the amelodentine junction; in Type II the height is at least % of normal height, in Type III its height is below % of normal and Type IV shows no bone continuity and indicates total failure of the technique (TRINDADE *et al,* 2005)(SHARMA et *al,* 2012).

Periapical radiographs were taken by positioning the film on the palatal surface in the canine region, with its long axis parallel to the long axis of this unit. The central x-ray beam was directed towards the canine eminence and its head was positioned on the distal and inferior edge of the nasal wing. This positioning has been standardised using radiographic positioners to achieve greater parallelism. All x-ray exposure risks were minimised through the use of lead shields.

The X-rays were assessed in a dimly lit area using a negatoscope and an assessment guide made from acetate paper. As a reference for the examiner of the level of bone gain, the coverage of the root surfaces of the teeth adjacent to the cleft was used; the presence or absence of the canine or supernumerary elements had no influence on the analysis of the data. Each examiner assessed the examination separately and differences were resolved by reviewing the cases (TRINDADE *et al*, 2005).

Evaluating the radiographic success and failure criteria, success was considered when the height of the bone formed at the cleft site was classified as I or II according to the Bergland scale. The clinical criteria helped to guide and correlate the findings, such as the presence of a fistula, with the radiographic presentations.

Although pattern III maintained maxillary bone continuity and favoured complete closure of the oral-nasal communication, it does not favour subsequent dental rehabilitation and orthodontic treatment. Thus, the partial gains obtained by alveolar reconstruction do not characterise the absolute success of the surgical procedure (CARLINI et *al*, 2000)(TRINDADE et *al*, 2005) (SHARMA et *al*, 2012).

4.3.1 Analysing the data

The database was created using the MS EXCEL spreadsheet and analysed using the R statistical package version 3.2.5. Descriptive analysis was carried out by calculating absolute and relative frequencies. In order to verify associations between study variables and surgical success, we used the Chi-Square test or Fisher's Exact test. The significance

level adopted for this study was 5%.

CHAPTER 5

RESULTS:

A total of 53 patients were assessed, of whom 20 (37.7%) were female and 33 (62.3%) male. Most of them were over 12 years old, 58.5%, and 41.5% under 12 years old. A total of 19 (35.8%) were from the capital of Bahia itself and 34 (64.2%) from the interior **(Table D)**.

Table 1. Epidemiological Data of the Population

Variables	n=53	%
Gender		
Female	20	37,7
Male	33	62,3
Age group (years)		
Less than equal to 12	22	41,5
Greater than 12	31	58,5
Origin		
Capital	19	35,8
Inside	34	64,2

According to the type of cleft, 8 (15.1%) of the cases were complete bilateral. There were 15 (28.3%) complete unilateral clefts on the right and 24 (45.3%) on the left, which was the most frequent type. Incomplete unilateral clefts, the least frequent type, occurred on the right in only one case (1.9%) and on the left in 5 cases (9.4%) **(Table 2).**

The grafting time ranged from 12 to 24 months. There were 25 (47.2 per cent) of them in the 12 to 18 month range and the remaining 28 (52.8 per cent) in the 19 to 24 month range. During the revision appointments, the presence of an infectious process was found in 12 (22.6%) patients, the reapproach rate was 15.1% (8 patients) and the presence of a

fistula was detected in 3 (5.7%) of the **cases (Table 2).**

Post-operative oral hygiene was classified as satisfactory in 31 (58.5%), regular in

19 (35.8%) and unsatisfactory in 3 (5.7%). The predominant radiographic type was type II

with 24 (45.3%) of the cases, followed by type I with 16 (30.2%) and type III with 11 (20.8%).

Type IV, which characterises the complete loss of the graft, had a rate of 3.8%, a total of

only 2 cases **(Table 2).**

Table 2. Characteristics of the Study Population

Variables	n=53	%
Type of crack		
Full bilateral	8	15,1
Unilateral full right	15	28,3
Unilateral full left	24	45,3
Unilateral incomplete right	1	1,9
Unilateral incomplete left	5	9,4
Grafting time (months)		
12a 18	25	47,2
19 a 24	28	52,8
Hygiene		
Unsatisfactory	3	5,7
Regular	19	35,8
Satisfactory	31	58,5
Infection		
Yes	12	22,6
No	41	77,4
Re-approach		
Yes	8	15,1
No	45	84,9
Fistula		
Yes	3	5,7
No	50	94,3
Radiographic type		
I	16	30,2
II	24	45,3
III	11	20,8
IV	2	3,8

The radiographic aspects classified as Type I and II were considered to be successful

and, consequently, Type III and IV as unsuccessful. This shows a high success rate with a

percentage of 75.5 %. **(Graph 1)**

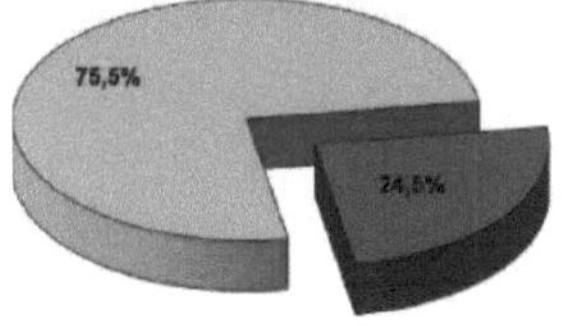

Graph 1. Success Rate

Significant associations with procedural success were identified depending on age group (p<0.001). Patients under the age of 12 had a 100 per cent success rate, while those over 12 had a success rate of only 58.1 per cent.

The type of cleft was also associated with surgical success (p=0.010). Complete bilateral clefts had a success rate of only 37.5 per cent, while unilateral clefts had high rates. The right complete cleft had a 93.3% success rate and the left complete cleft had a 75.5% success rate. The incomplete one on the left was 100% successful. The only case of incomplete right was a failure **(Table 3).**

The variables Grafting time and Hygiene were not associated with surgical success (p=0.933 and p=0.495). The percentages of success in
in terms of grafting time are very close. With regard to the degree of hygiene, the difference between the percentages of success between those classified as unsatisfactory (66.7%) and regular (68.4%) is irrelevant. In the sample group with satisfactory hygiene, the percentage of success was 80.0%, but this difference was not statistically significant.

Table 3. Statistical Correlation of the Data Found

Variables	Surgical success		
	n=40	75,5 %	p-value
Age group (years)			**<0,001**
Less than equal to 12	22	100,0	

Greater than 12	18	58,1	
Type of crack			**0,010**
Full bilateral	3	37,5	
Unilateral full right	14	93,3	
Unilateral full left	18	75,5	
Unilateral incomplete right	0	0,0	
Unilateral incomplete left	5	100,0	
Grafting time (months)			
12a 18			0,933
19 a 24	19	76,0	
	21	75,0	
Hygiene			0,495
Unsatisfactory	2	66,7	
Regular	13	68,4	
Satisfactory		80,0	

CHAPTER 6

DISCUSSION:

In this series of cases, there was a slight predominance of male patients, which is in line with the literature, which shows a prevalence of 60 to 80 % of cases (OWENS *et al*, 1985)(LOFFREDO et *al*, 1994) (PALOMINA et *al*, 2000)(CUNHA et *al*, 2004). Regarding the type and extent of the cleft, there was a predominance of complete cleft lip and palate in the cases studied. These findings were also confirmed by Freitas et al. in 2004.

Another epidemiological study carried out in Minas Gerais traced the profile of clefts in a specialised centre in Belo Horizonte. Its sample comprised 1219 patients who were registered between 2005 and 2008. Of this total, 49% had a transforamen incisor cleft, 26% post-foramen, 19% pre-foramen and 3% other types of malformations. The interior of the state had the highest number of members with 38.5% of all cases (DI NINNO et *al*, 2010). These figures are in line with the research carried out, which showed a majority of transforaminal clefts and identified a greater demand for patients in the interior of the state.

With regard to laterality, the majority of clefts were located on the left, followed by the right and bilateral. Left-sided unilateral clefts are more frequent than right-sided ones, which in turn are more frequent than bilateral ones, and it has even been stated that left-sided clefts may be 1.6 times more frequent than right-sided ones. There is still no plausible explanation for this differentiation. It is believed that, at the beginning of pregnancy, there is a greater blood supply to the right side of the foetus due to greater blood pressure in the right internal carotid artery (FREITAS *et al*, 2004)(CERQUEIRA *et al*, 2005). This study takes into account the fact that patients who underwent premaxillary repositioning were excluded and therefore had complete bilateral transforaminal cleft lip and palate, which reduced this type of sample.

Correlating the success rate of alveolar grafting with the age of the patients, a study by Tabrizi et al (2013) compared two groups with different age ranges. Their results showed that the group with the lowest age range, between 9 and 12 years, had the highest success rate with a percentage of 92%, while the second group achieved only 20%. These results corroborate those found in this study, as a 100 per cent success rate was achieved in the group of patients under 12.

Another study analysing the success rate of 104 patients undergoing secondary alveolar bone grafting at the Hospital Sant Joan de Déu (HSJD) in Barcelona found no statistical difference in relation to age. With a mean age of 14.45 years, he obtained a total of 100 (96.2%) successful cases. As he had a good success rate, he could not relate his failure to age. This study showed that even in young patients, success with autogenous iliac crest grafts is high. Although the ideal time to perform it is before the eruption of the permanent canine, its potential for incorporation is high. However, what we see in the literature is that the later the rehabilitation, the more obscure the prognosis (LUQUE-MARTIN *et al,* 2013).

According to a recent study that assessed the predictors associated with complications in graft surgery, the need for the surgery to be repeated due to failure was associated with post-surgical complications, the patient's age, gender and the type of cleft. Reoperation also resulted in the formation of more scar tissue and in the future could compromise local blood supply and the healing of soft and hard tissues (PESSOA et *al,* 2015).

Patients with bilateral clefts were significantly more likely to have complications during graft surgery. Patients with bilateral transforaminal clefts were more likely to have to have the surgery redone, as well as a tendency to have more complications than those with unilateral clefts. Tertiary grafts have also not shown the same success rates as secondary grafts (MENDONÇA et *al*, 2011)(LUQUE-MARTIN et *al*, 2014).

Although most studies point to the autogenous graft with iliac Christian as the best option for alveolar reconstructions due to its good quantity and the supply of medullary and cortical material, some studies believe that the removal of the graft from the iliac bone has been the subject of controversy. The post-operative complications that can occur with the patient, such as persistent pain, haemorrhage, visible scarring, lengthy recovery time, injury to the femoral cutaneous nerve, pelvic fracture and peritonitis (PESSOA *et al*, 2015).

New technologies, such as BMP, are being used with the aim of finding an alternative to the use of autogenous bone; however, no new technique can be considered superior to the traditional bone graft taken from the iliac crest. In addition, more safety studies with regard to oncogenetic potential are needed, especially for use in childhood (CHEN et *al*, 2004)(PESSOA et *al*, 2015).

Radiographically, the study by Trindade et al. (2005) assessed bone formation in the alveolar fissure region after a minimum of 2 years post-operative secondary alveolar grafting. Carrying out the procedure on patients aged between 9 and 12 and using the Berland scale as a parameter, they found a rate of 71% type I bone and 14% type II. Compared to the findings of this study, it can be seen that despite the age factor being present, 45.3% of type II bone height and 30.2% of type I bone height were obtained, both considered successes.

Sharma et al. in 2012, using the same radiographic scores and evaluating a total of 10 patients, found type I bone formation in 7 cases (87.5%) after 6 months of radiographic follow-up. They found one case of no bone formation (type IV) in a patient with a complete bilateral cleft. Demonstrating a small sample and limited follow-up time, a high rate of type I formation was observed. Studies show that bone resorption at the grafting site remains active for up to one year post-operatively. In the cases reported in

research, there was a follow-up time of one to two years and it can be concluded that after this period the correlation between success and time is no longer statistically significant.

Another study using the same classification table evaluated 129 patients with cleft lip and palate. They obtained a success rate of 79.1% (101 cases), with no statistical difference in relation to the age factor. However, they observed that patients aged between 9 and 12 had a higher success rate with greater height of bone formation. On the other hand, individuals aged 14 and over had worse results, with only 3 out of 8 in the study being in the success range established by the study (OPITZ *et al,* 1999).

The data found an incidence of 3.8% of cases with type IV bone. This type of assessment is related to the lack of bone formation at the cleft site and the need for reoperation. On the other hand, 8 cases required a new surgical procedure, 1 due to the formation of a fistula and 5 due to recurrent infectious processes with the formation of bone sequestration and partial loss of the graft. These data, in comparison with those described in the literature, relate to patients who need tertiary grafts, so the age group contributes greatly to the rate of reoperation. (MENDONÇA et *al,* 2011)(LUQUE-MARTIN et *al,* 2014)(PESSOA et *al,* 2015).

Routine radiographic examination has many limiting factors, such as image magnification and distortion, overlapping structures, a limited number of identifiable reference points and positioning problems, all of which can adversely affect image quality. There are also obvious shortcomings in trying to obtain three-dimensional information from a two-dimensional image. With the use of cone beam computed tomography, the aforementioned problems can be avoided (LEITE *et al,* 2014).

The alveolar cleft has traditionally been studied using conventional two-dimensional examinations, such as periapical, occlusal and panoramic radiographs. However, 2D images of a three-dimensional bone defect do not allow the volume of the alveolar cleft to be measured. These images only measure bone height, as they do not show the depth of the alveolar cleft, and the professional is often faced with a defect that is larger than initially planned, which makes the prognosis of the surgery difficult, as the cleft must be completely sealed. Pre-surgical volumetric quantification of the defect is of great value, as it determines the amount of graft material needed for the procedure. In addition, post-surgical monitoring with 3D scans is useful for orthodontic and prosthetic treatments to determine orthodontic movement and implant placement (LEITE et *al,* 2014).

CHAPTER 7

CONCLUSION:

Thus, the alveolar grafts carried out at the reference centre of Hospital Santo Antônio (Obras Sociais Irmã Dulce) - Centrinho, following the philosophy of the Craniofacial Anomaly Rehabilitation Hospital of the University of São Paulo (HRAC-UUSP), have been achieving a success rate similar to that found in the literature.

The predictability found in secondary alveolar grafts using the iliac crest as a donor area makes this procedure the one of choice to be applied routinely in the service.

The biggest statistically significant factor in achieving a high success rate is age. As advocated in the literature, patients who undergo cleft repair early have a better prognosis than those who start in the tertiary phase. Although oral hygiene and infection contribute to the prognosis, they are correlated with local management and post-operative care.

It is therefore necessary to use more and more studies to assess the quality of service provision. The use of computerised tomography helps and provides an accurate diagnosis of the need found in the treatment of this population.

Expanding biomaterial options is also necessary. The promising use of RhBMP-2 in patients who need tertiary alveolar grafting, achieving good bone filling results, should be encouraged through research into its use in the Unified Health Service (SUS).

CHAPTER 8

BIBLIOGRAPHICAL REFERENCES:

1- CARLINI JL.; ZÉTOLA AL.; SOUZA RP. de, *et al.* Autogenous iliac Christian graft in the reconstruction of the alveolar process in cleft patients

labiopalatine - Study of 30 cases. **Rev Col Bras Cirur.** v.27, n.6,p.389-383. 2000.

2- COUTINHO ALF.; LIMA M de C.; KITAMURA MAP, *et al.* Epidemiological profile of patients with orofacial clefts treated at a reference centre in northeastern Brazil. **Rev Bras Saúde Matern Infant.** v.9, n.2, p. 149-156. 2009.

3- SILVA FILHO, OG.; FREITAS, JAS. Morphological characterisation and embryological origin. IN: TRINDADE, IEK.; SILVA FILHO, OG. **Cleft lip and palate.** São Paulo: Santos, 2007. chap. 2, p. 17-49.

4- LE BT.; WOO I. Alveolar cleft repair in adults using guided bone regeneration with mineralised allograft for dental implant site development: A report of 2 cases. J **Oral Maxillofac Surg.** v.67, p.1716-1722. 2009.

5- BRYDON CA.; CONWAY J.; KLING R, et *al.* Cleft lip and/or palate: One organisation's experience with more than a quarter million surgeries during the past decade. The **J of Craniofac Surg.** v.25,n.5,p. 1601 -609. 2014.

6- SEKHON PS.; ETHUNANDAN M.; MARKUS AF, et *al.* Congenital anomalies associated with cleft lip and palate - An analysis of 1623 consecutive patients. **Cleft Palate-Craniofac J.** v.48, n.4, p.371-378. 2011.

7- BORBA AM.; BORGES AH.; SILVA CSV da, et *al.* Predictors of complication for alveolar cleft bone graft. **Brit J of Oral and Maxillofac Surg.** v.52, p. 174-178. 2014.

8- FREITAS JA de S.; GARIB DG.; TRINDADE-SUEDAM IK, et *al.* Rehabilitative treatment of cleft lip and palate: Experience of the Hospital for Rehabilitation of Craniofacial Anomalies - USP (HRAC-USP) - Part. 3: Oral and Maxillofacial Surgery . J **Appl Oral Sei.** v.20, n.6, p.673-679. 2012.

9- PRECIOUS DS. A new reliable method for alveolar bone grafting at about 6 years of age. **Am J Ass of Oral Maxillofac Surg.** v.67, p.2045-2053. 2009.

10-SANTIAGO PE.; SCHUSTER LA.; LEVY-BERCOWSKI D. Management of the alveolar cleft. **Clin Plastic Surg.** v.41, p.219-232. 2014.

11- HALL HD.; POSNICK JC. Early results of secondary bone grafts in 106 alveolar clefts. J **Oral Maxillofac Surg.** v.41, p.289-294. 1983.

12-KAZEMI A.; STEARNS JW.; FONSECA RJ. Secondary grafting in the alveolar cleft patient. **Am N Clin Oral Maxillofac Surg.** v.14, p.477-490. 2002.

13- THUAKSUBAM N.; NUNTANARANONT T.; PRIPATNANONT P. A comparison of autogenous bone graft combined with deproteinised bovine bone and autogenous bone graft alone for treatment of alveolar cleft. **J of Oral Maxillofac Surg.** v.39, p.1175-1180. 2010.

14-MOORE KL. Clinical Embryology. Guanabara, 1990.

15-SILVA RS dos S. Cleft lip and palate. Centre for Specialisation in Clinical Speech Therapy - Oral Motricity. Rio de Janeiro, 1999. 36 p.

16-AVERY, JK. Development of the face and palate. In: AVERY, JK. Fundamentals of oral histology and embryology: a clinical approach. 2. ed. Rio de Janeiro: Guanabara Koogan, 2001. Chap. 4, p. 38-47

17-MOORE, KL.; PERSAUD, TVN. Clinical embryology. Rio de Janeiro: Elsevier, 2008.

18-CERQUEIRA MN, et al. Occurrence of Cleft Lip and Palate in the City of São José dos Campos - SP. **Rev Bras Epidemiol.** v. 8, n. 2, p. 161-166. 2005.

19-ESCOFFIÉ-RAMIREZ, M. et al. Association of cleft lip and/or palate with socioeconomic position variables: a study of cases and controls. **Rev Bras Saúde Mater Infant,** Recife, v.10, n.3, p. 323-329, july/sept. 2010.

20-GARIB, DG. et al. Etiology of malocclusions: clinical perspective (part III) - cleft lip and palate. **Rev Clin Ortod Dental Press,** Maringá, v.9, n.4, p. 30- 36. 2010.

21-BARONEZA JE.; FARIA MJSS. de; KUASNE H, *et al.* Epidemiological data of patients with cleft lip and palate in a specialised institution in Londrina, Paraná State. **Maringá,** v.27, n1, p.31-35. 2005.

22-FIGUEIREDO, MC. et al. Complete unilateral cleft lip and palate: dental alterations and malocclusion - clinical case report. RFO, **Porto Alegre,** v.13, n.3, p. 73-77. 2008.

23-ZAMBONATO, TCF. et al. Profile of hearing aid users with cleft lip and palate. **Braz. J. Otorhinolaryngol.,** v.75, n.6, p. 888-892. 2009.

24-MASTRANTONIO, SS.; CASTILHO, ARF. de; GARRARA, CFC. Dental anomalies in children with cleft lip and palate. **Odontol clín-cient., Recife,** v.8, n.3, p. 273-278. 2009.

25-KHAN, M., et al. A revised classification of the cleft lip and palate. T **Canadian J of Plast Surg,** v. 21, n. 1, p. 48-50. 2013.

26- KERNAHAN, da; STARK, RB. A new classification for cleft lip and cleft palate. **Plast Reconstr Surg.** v. 22, p. 435. 1958.

27-SPINA, VA. Proposed modification for the classification of cleft lip and cleft palate. **Cleft palate J;** v. 10, p. 251. 1974.

28- BRUNER, G. et al. Prevalence of lip and palate cleft in Rio Claro - SP, from 2006 to 2009. **Odontol Clín Cient.,** v. 11, n. 2, p. 117-119. 2012.

29-SHKOUKANI, M., et al. (2013). Cleft lip - a comprehensive review. [Online]. Available at <http://doi:3389/fped.2013.00053> [Accessed 17/06/2015],

30- TUJI, F., et al. (2009). Multidisciplinary treatment in the rehabilitation of patients with cleft lip and/or palate in a public hospital. Revista Paraense de Medicina, 23(2).

31-LURENTT, K., et al. Orthognathic surgery in a patient with cleft lip and palate. Case report. **Rev Cir Traumatol Buco-Maxilo-Fac,** v.12, n. 1, pp.47-52. 2012

32-RASPALL, G. Maxillofacial surgery. Madrid, Editorial Médica Panamericana S.A, pp. 39-44. 1997.

33-ANNASTASSOV, G., JOOS, U. Comprehensive Management of cleft lip and palate deformities. **J Oral and Maxillofac Surg,** v. 59, p. 1062-1075. 2001.

34-AMORIM, J. Comparative study of the von langenbeck, veau-wardill-kilner and furlow palatoplasty techniques. University of Porto Faculty of Medicine. Arquivos de Medicina, v. 28, n. 2, p. 36-43. 2014

35-ANDERSEN K, et al. Donor site morbidity after reconstruction of alveolar bone defects with mandibular symphyseal bone grafts in cleft patients - 111 consecutive patients. **Int J Oral Maxillofac Surg;** v. 43, p. 428-432. 2014.

36-KON KS. et al. Treatment algorithm for bilateral alveolar cleft based on the position of the premaxilla and the width of the alveolar gap. **J of Plast Reconstr and Aesthet Surg,** v. 66, p. 1212-1218. 2013.

37-BOYNE PJ.; SANDS NR. Secondary bone grafting of residual alveolar and palate cleft. J Oral Surg. v. 30, p.87-92, 1972.

38- SILVA FILHO, O.G.; FERRARI JÚNIOR, F.M.; ROCHA, D.L. et al. Classification of cleft lip and palate: brief history, clinical considerations and suggested modifications. *Rev Bras Cir,* v.82, p.59-65, 1992.

39-RIBEIRO, Alexandre de Almeida; LEAL, Luíse; THUIN, Rawlson de. Morphological analysis of cleft lip and palate patients at the Craniofacial Anomalies Treatment Centre of the State of Rio de Janeiro. Rev. **Dent. Press Ortodon. Ortop. Facial,**

Maringá , v. 12, n. 5, p. 109-118, Oct. 2007 .

40-LIMA, M. L. S. et al. Cleft lip and palate - Considerations on interdisciplinary treatment. Orthodont Science and Practice, v.1, n.2, p. 173-177, 2008.

41-MENDONÇA, JCG; LIMA COSTA, CM; TERRA, GAP. Use of autogenous bone graft from the iliac crest in the reconstruction of an alveolar cleft in a patient cleft: case report. **Rev Bras Cir Craniomaxillofac.,** v. 14, n. 3, p. 162165. 2011.

42-BRASIL. Ministry of Health. Portaria n° 62 SAS/MS, de 19 de abril de 1994, Dispõe normas para o cadastramento de hospitais que realizadas procedimentos integrados para reabilitação de portadores de fissuras lábio-palatal para o SUS. Federal Official Gazette, Brasilia, 1994.

43-TAI CC.; SUTHERLAND IS.; MCFADDEN L. Prospective analysis of secondary alveolar bone grafting using computed tomography. **J Oral Maxillofac Surg.** v. 58, n. 11, p. 1241 -1249, Nov. 2000.

44-FEICHTINGER M.; MOSSBOCK R.; KARCHER H. Evaluation of bone volume following nobe grafting in patients with unilateral clefts of lip, alveolus and palate using a CT-guided three-dimensional navigation system . J **Craniomaxillofac Surg.** v.34,p.144-149.Mar. 2006.

45-LUQUE-MARTIN E.; TOBELLA-CAMPS ML.; RIVERA-BARÓ A. Alveolar graft in the cleft lip and palate patient: Review of 104 cases. **Med Oral Pathol Oral Cir Bucal,** v.19, n.5, p.531-537.Sep. 2014.

46-TABRIZI R.; ZAMIRI B.; DANESTE H.; ARABION H. Outcome of bone availability after secondary alveolar bone graft in two age groups. **The J of Craniofac Surg.** v.24, n.6, p.565-567.Mar. 2013.

47-NIGHTINGALE C.; WITHEROW H.; REID FDA, *et al.* Comparative reproducibility of three methods of radiographic assessment of alveolar bone grafting. **Euro J of Ortho.**

v.25, p.35-41.2003.

48-TRINDADE IK.; MAZZOTTINI R.; SILVA FILHO OG da, et al. Long-Term radiographic assessment of secondary alveolar bone grafting outcomes in patients with alveolar clefts. **Oral Surg Oral Med Oral Pathol Oral Radiol Endod,** v. 1, n. 7, p. 100-127, Sept. 2005.

49-SHARMA S., *et al.* Secondary alveolar bone grafting: Radiographic and clinical evaluation. **An of Maxillofac Surg.** v. 2, n. 1, p. 41 -45. Jan/Jun. 2012.

50- LEITE, TB; BEZERRA, BT; SILVA, LCF da. Volumetric quantification of the alveolar cleft in cleft patients. Rev. Cir. Traumatol. v. 14, n. 2, p. 103-108.2014.

51-DI NINNO CQ. de MS.; FONSECA LFN.; PIMENTA MVE, et *al.* Epidemiological survey of patients with cleft lip and/or palate at a specialised centre in Belo Horizonte. Rev CEFAC. v.27, n.1, p.19-22. Dec. 2010 - POR NA DISCUSSÃO.

52- Nazer J, Hubner ME, Catalán M. Incidence of cleft lip and palate in the Maternidad Del Holpital Clínico de la Universidad de Chile and in Chilean maternity hospitals participating in the Estudio Colaborativo Latino Americano de Malformaciones Congénitas (ECLAMC). Rev Méd Chile. 2001; 129: 285-93...

53- Loffredo LCM, Souza JMP, Yunes J, Freitas JAS, Spiri WC. Cleft lip: case-control study. Rev Saúde Pública. 1994; 28: 213-7.

54- Cunha ECM, Fontana R, Fontana T, Silva WR, Moreira QVP, Garcias GL, Roth MGM. Anthropometry and risk factors in newborns with facial clefts. Rev Bras Epidemiol. 2004; 7: 417-22

55- Palomino H, Guzmán E, Blanco R. Familial recurrence of cleft lip with or without velopalatine fissure of non-syndromic origin in Chilean populations. Rev Méd Chile. 2000; 128: 286-93.

56-Owens JR, Jones JW, Harris F. Epidemiology of facial clefting. Arc Dis Child. 1985;

60: 521-4.

57- . Freitas JAS, Dalben GS, Santamaria Júnior M, Freitas PZ. Current information on the characterisation of orofacial clefts in Brazil. Braz. Oral Res. 2004; 18: 128-33. 19. Magdalenic-Mestrovic M, Bagatin M. An epidemiological study of orofacial clefts in Croatia 1988-1998. J Craniomaxillofac Surg. 2005; 33: 85-90

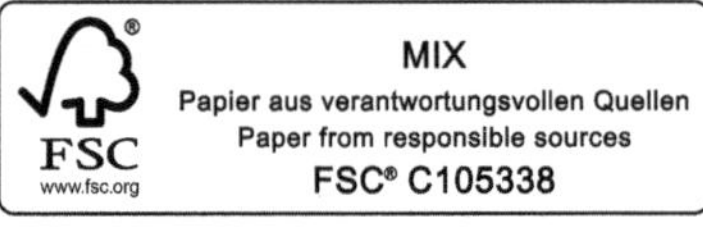

Printed by Books on Demand GmbH, Norderstedt / Germany